1

QUIT CRAVINGS:
The sneaky method

By

Neville lawson

CONTENTS

Part IV: Strategies for Substitution

Part V: Moderation and Balance

Part VI: Conquering Particular Wants

Part VII: Developing a Supportive Environment

Part VIII: Upkeep and Extended Prosperity

Part IX. Conclusion.

DISCLAIMER

The information provided in this book is for general informational purposes only. It is meant as a complement to enhance the reader's understanding.

or retained without approval from the publisher or creator.

Introduction

Fighting excess weight has become a constant struggle for millions of people in a world where the prevalence of obesity is rising unabatedly. Cravings are the sneaky enemy at the center of this battle. We indulge in unhealthy foods as a result of these constant cravings, which are frequently overwhelming and irresistible. This leads to a vicious cycle of overeating and weight gain.

What if we could, however, take back control over our cravings and create a route that leads to long-term wellness and weight loss? Welcome to "QUIT CRAVINGS: The Sneaky method."

With the help of this ground-breaking book, we will go beyond the confines of conventional dieting paradigms and explore the psychology, physiology, and useful techniques associated with overcoming cravings. We'll examine the revolutionary potential of tackling cravings at their core, revealing the secret to long-term weight control and enhanced general health, by drawing on the most recent research, individual experiences, and real-world success stories.

As you read this book, you'll learn that the key to overcoming cravings isn't deprivation or sheer willpower, but rather identifying a behind method—an alternate strategy that places an emphasis on moderation, mindfulness, and substitute. Gaining the knowledge and self-assurance required to skillfully negotiate the intricate terrain of food cravings with grace and resilience will enable you to identify the triggers and mechanisms behind your cravings and put targeted strategies in place to counter them.

"QUIT CRAVINGS" is a manifesto for regaining your agency, developing self-awareness, and creating a healthy relationship with food and body, though it is more than just a weight loss guide. It involves committing to a balanced, nourishing, and self-care lifestyle that values your mental, emotional, and spiritual health.

Recognize that you have company on this life-changing adventure. This book is your reliable companion—a ray of hope and direction in the turbulent sea of dietary confusion—whether you're fighting sugar cravings, struggling with emotional eating, or trying to find comfort from the allure of unhealthy foods.

Come along with me as we set out on a journey of self-awareness and empowerment. One conscious bite at a time, together we'll uncover the mysteries of kicking cravings, changing your body, and regaining your health.

overview of the obesity epidemic and the role of cravings

The modern era has brought about unprecedented progress in technology, medicine, and quality of life. Obesity, on the other hand, has become a silent epidemic that is still plaguing societies worldwide. Obesity, defined as the excessive accumulation of body fat, has emerged as one of the most pressing public health concerns of the twenty-first century.

Obesity is a complex medical condition with far-reaching consequences for physical and psychological well-being. Its prevalence has risen dramatically in recent decades, with alarming rates reported across all age groups, genders, and geographic regions. Obesity rates have nearly tripled globally since 1975, with more than 650 million adults classified as obese in 2016.

The ramifications of this epidemic are significant. Obesity significantly increases the risk of developing a wide range of chronic diseases, including type 2 diabetes, cardiovascular disease, certain cancers, and musculoskeletal disorders. Furthermore, it places a heavy burden on healthcare systems, resulting in skyrocketing healthcare costs and a lower quality of life for affected people.

At the heart of the obesity epidemic is a fundamental aspect of human physiology and behavior: cravings. Cravings, which are intense desires for specific foods, play an important role in promoting overeating and weight gain. They are not whims or passing fancies, but strong urges that are deeply ingrained in our biological and psychological makeup.

Understanding the mechanisms underlying cravings is critical for navigating the complexities of obesity. Genetic predisposition, hormonal imbalances, psychological stressors, environmental cues, and cultural influences all play a role in shaping cravings. In today's obesogenic environment, which is characterized by ubiquitous access to calorie-dense, highly palatable foods, these factors combine to fuel a vicious cycle of overconsumption and obesity.

Cravings occur on multiple levels, involving both the body and the mind. Cravings are mediated by intricate neural circuits in the brain's reward system that release neurotransmitters such as dopamine in response to the consumption of pleasurable foods. This neurochemical response reinforces the behavior, resulting in repeated bouts of overeating and addictive patterns similar to substance abuse.

A variety of psychological factors influence cravings, including emotional state, stress levels, learned behaviors, and social cues. Many people use food as a form of comfort or distraction, coping with negative emotions or relieving stress. Over time, these associations become deeply ingrained, making it difficult to break free from the emotional eating and craving cycle.

In essence, cravings are a major impediment to successful weight management and a major cause of the obesity epidemic. To address cravings, a multifaceted approach is required, encompassing biological, psychological, social, and environmental factors. Individuals can regain control of their eating habits, achieve long-term weight loss, and improve their overall health and well-being by understanding the root causes of cravings and implementing targeted strategies to reduce their impact.

Outlining the Idea of "Quitting Cravings"

The concept of "quitting cravings" may seem unattainable in a world where temptations appear everywhere and our eating habits are largely determined by our cravings. But what if I told you that it is both feasible and within your reach?

Welcome to the revolutionary idea of "quitting cravings"—a mentality-shifting idea that gives you the ability to reclaim your relationship with food and free yourself from the chains of incessant needs.

Fundamentally, "giving up cravings" is about taking back control of your eating habits and freeing yourself from the oppressive grip of constant cravings for bad foods. It's important to understand that cravings are learned patterns of behavior that can be broken and replaced with healthier ones; they are neither inevitable nor unbeatable.

But first, why should you even think about giving up cravings? The impact that cravings can have on your overall health, happiness, and quality of life is the key to the solution. Cravings have a negative impact on the body and the psyche, as they can lead to weight gain and obesity, encourage compulsive eating, and exacerbate chronic illnesses.

You start a life-changing path toward increased vitality, empowerment, and self-awareness when you accept the idea of giving up cravings. Saying "yes" to a life of balance, mindfulness, and abundance is more important than merely saying "no" to alluring treats or depriving oneself of pleasure.

We'll examine the root causes of cravings, dispel myths, and present research-backed methods for conquering them throughout this book. There are a plethora of tools and techniques available to assist you in permanently eliminating cravings, ranging from reprogramming your brain's reward system to understanding the psychological triggers behind cravings and developing healthier habits.

Perhaps most importantly, though, is that overcoming cravings is a shared community effort motivated by a common commitment to wellness and health, rather than an isolated undertaking. Be it resisting sugar cravings, overcoming emotional eating, or overcoming a food addiction, remember that support exists. In unison, we shall surmount obstacles, commemorate accomplishments, and enable one another to lead the most abundant and lively lives possible.

Is it now your time to take this life-changing adventure? Ready to take back mastery over your cravings and open the door to a more contented, healthier version of yourself? If so, let's get started and explore the fascinating world of overcoming cravings. This is the beginning of your journey.

Personal anecdotes or testimonials about overcoming cravings and weight loss

1. Sarah's Story: Breaking Free From Emotional Eating

For years, Sarah was trapped in a vicious cycle of emotional eating. When she was stressed or anxious, she turned to sugary snacks and comfort foods for relief, only to be left feeling guilty and ashamed later.

Her weight steadily increased, and despite numerous attempts to diet, she was unable to break free from the grip of cravings.

But everything changed when Sarah discovered the benefits of mindfulness and self-compassion. She learned to identify the underlying emotions driving her cravings through therapy and support groups, and she developed healthier coping mechanisms to deal with them. Instead of turning to food for comfort, she found solace in activities such as journaling, meditation, and being outside.

Sarah noticed a significant change in her relationship with food as she gained a better understanding of her triggers and learned to respond to them with kindness rather than judgment. Cravings no longer controlled her, and she felt empowered to make nourishing choices that supported her health and well-being. She gradually lost weight naturally, not through deprivation or strict dieting, but through a renewed sense of self-awareness and self-care.

Sarah is now living proof that it is possible to break the cycle of emotional eating and lose weight for good. She transformed her relationship with food and regained control of her cravings by practicing mindfulness and self-compassion, paving the way for a healthier, happier life.

2. Mark's Journey: Overcoming the Desire for Late-Night Snacking

Mark had struggled with late-night cravings for as long as he could remember, which sabotaged his weight loss efforts. After a long day at work, he found himself reaching for salty snacks and sugary treats to relax, frequently devouring entire bags of chips or containers of ice cream in one sitting. Despite his best intentions to eat healthily, he couldn't shake the allure of late-night indulgence.

Mark was determined to break the cycle and took a different approach. Instead of fighting his cravings, he focused on understanding the underlying causes.

Through introspection and self-reflection, he realized that his late-night snacking was motivated by boredom and stress, rather than hunger.

Armed with this knowledge, Mark began implementing targeted strategies to confront his cravings. He replaced unhealthy snacks with healthier options like air-popped popcorn, sliced vegetables with hummus, and Greek yogurt with fruit. He also developed a relaxing bedtime routine to help him unwind and de-stress before sleeping, which included activities such as reading, taking a warm bath, and practicing deep breathing exercises.

Mark gradually began to notice a significant change in his nighttime habits. The desire to snack mindlessly subsided, and he felt more satisfied and content with his healthier choices. He gradually lost excess weight and gained new energy and vitality, all without depriving himself or succumbing to feelings of guilt or shame.

Mark's journey is a powerful reminder that with patience, persistence, and self-awareness, it is possible to overcome even the most tenacious cravings and achieve long-term weight loss success. By addressing the underlying triggers and adopting healthier habits, he has transformed his relationship with food and reclaimed control over his health and wellbeing.

Objectives and Goals:

"QUIT CRAVINGS: The Sneaky Method" aims to give readers a thorough manual on how to overcome cravings and achieve long-term weight loss using a distinct, all-encompassing strategy. The book intends to empower readers to take charge of their eating habits, enhance their relationship with food, and eventually reach their weight loss goals by addressing the underlying causes of cravings and providing useful strategies for managing them.

One of the book's main objectives is to inform readers about the biological, psychological, and environmental elements that underlie cravings. Readers will be better able to identify and effectively deal with their cravings by developing awareness and understanding.

2. Provide Useful Strategies:

" Quit Cravings" offers a plethora of tactics and methods based on research for controlling cravings in day-to-day living. Readers will learn a variety of tools to help them overcome cravings and make healthier food choices, from mindfulness practices and substitution strategies to moderation techniques and creating a supportive environment.

3. Encourage Sustainable Weight Loss:

The book advocates for a sustainable weight loss strategy that emphasizes long-term behavior change rather than short-term diets or quick fixes. Readers will learn how to develop enduring habits that promote their health and well-being by using the back door approach, which emphasizes mindfulness, moderation, and substitution.

4. Promote Empowerment:
" Quit Cravings" aims to empower readers to take charge of their journey to successful weight loss by highlighting the significance of self-awareness, self-compassion, and self-efficacy. Readers will be encouraged to believe in their own ability to conquer cravings and accomplish their goals through stories from personal experience, endorsements, and useful exercises.

5. Offer Support and Guidance: Understanding that kicking cravings can be difficult, the book attempts to give readers the encouragement and direction they require to remain resilient and driven. Readers will discover a multitude of tools to assist them in staying on course, whether it is through advice on handling social situations, building a network of support, or handling setbacks.

In the end, " Quit Cravings " is a guide to a happier, healthier life free from the hold of cravings rather than merely a book on weight loss. Through adopting the sneaky method strategy and practicing self-compassion, moderation, and mindfulness, readers will find a new way to take charge of their health and well-being and reach their weight loss objectives.

Part 1: Understanding Cravings.

What is craving?

Cravings are strong desires or urges for particular foods or flavors. Cravings, as opposed to regular hunger, which signals a general need for nourishment, are usually focused on specific types of foods that are high in sugar, salt, fat, or other satisfying qualities. Cravings can take the form of a strong desire to eat a specific food item or a persistent desire to consume particular flavors or textures.

Cravings frequently contain both psychological and physiological components. Emotions, environmental cues, or learned behaviors can all trigger cravings. Stress, boredom, and social situations, for example, can all trigger cravings, as can exposure to food-related cues like advertisements, smells, or visual stimuli. Furthermore, habits and associations formed over time can contribute to the development of cravings, resulting in automatic responses to specific situations or cues.

Physiologically, the body's hormonal and neurotransmitter systems can influence cravings. Hormones such as leptin, ghrelin, insulin, and cortisol regulate appetite, metabolism, and energy balance, which can affect cravings. Similarly, neurotransmitters such as dopamine, serotonin, and endorphins function in the brain's reward system and can influence cravings by reinforcing pleasurable eating experiences.

Cravings are a complex combination of biological, psychological, and environmental factors. While cravings can be intense and difficult to control at times, understanding the underlying causes and how to manage them effectively can help people make healthier food choices and maintain balanced eating habits.

The psychology behind cravings: triggers, habits, and emotions.

The psychology of cravings includes a number of factors, such as triggers, habits, and emotions, all of which interact to shape our desire for certain foods. Understanding these psychological mechanisms is essential for successfully managing cravings.

1. Triggers: Cravings are triggered by external or internal cues that activate associations or memories with specific foods. These triggers can range from environmental cues (such as the sight or smell of food) to emotional states (such as stress or boredom), social situations (such as gatherings or celebrations), and even specific times of day. For example, passing by a bakery and smelling freshly baked cookies may cause a craving for sweets, whereas feeling anxious before a presentation may cause a desire for comfort foods. Identifying and recognising these triggers is an important step in learning to control cravings.

2. Habits: Cravings are influenced by habits that shape and reinforce them. When we repeat a behavior (for example, reaching for a snack when stressed), it becomes ingrained as a habit, and cravings may arise automatically in response to certain cues or situations. Over time, these habits can become deeply entrenched and difficult to break. However, habits are malleable, and we can weaken the link between triggers and cravings by consciously reshaping our routines and responses. This could entail swapping unhealthy habits for healthier ones, such as going for a walk or practicing deep breathing instead of reaching for food when stressed.

3. Emotions: Cravings and emotions are often linked as food can provide comfort, pleasure, or distract from negative feelings. Emotional eating, or eating in response to emotions rather than hunger, is a common phenomenon that can lead to the development of cravings and unhealthy eating patterns. Emotional cravings are frequently triggered by specific emotions, such as stress, sadness, loneliness, or boredom, and can manifest as a desire for "comfort foods" that provide temporary relief or distraction.

Learning to recognize and address the underlying emotions that fuel cravings is critical for effective management. This could include finding alternative coping mechanisms for dealing with emotions, such as talking to a friend, practicing relaxation techniques, or participating in enjoyable activities that do not involve food.

To summarize, cravings are influenced by a complex interplay of triggers, habits, and emotions. Individuals can gain more control over their cravings and make healthier choices that benefit their overall well-being by understanding these psychological mechanisms and developing strategies to deal with them.

Physiological factors influencing cravings: hormones, neurotransmitters, and brain chemistry.

The physiological factors that influence cravings are inextricably linked to the intricate functioning of our hormonal systems, neurotransmitter activity, and brain chemistry. Understanding these biological mechanisms explains why cravings occur and how to manage them.

1. Hormones regulate hunger, satiety, and appetite, influencing food cravings.

Leptin, also known as the "satiety hormone," signals to the brain when we've had enough to eat, helping to suppress appetite and reduce cravings. Ghrelin, also known as the "hunger hormone," stimulates the appetite and promotes food intake, resulting in increased cravings. Furthermore, hormones such as insulin and cortisol can affect blood sugar levels and stress responses, influencing our desire for certain foods. Fluctuations or imbalances in these hormones can disrupt appetite regulation and contribute to cravings for specific foods, especially those high in sugar, salt, or fat.

2. **Neurotransmitters**: Neurotransmitters are chemical messengers in the brain that

affect physiological processes such as mood, cognition, and appetite. Dopamine, also known as the "pleasure neurotransmitter," is a key component of the brain's reward system, reinforcing behaviors associated with pleasure and motivation. When we consume highly palatable foods, such as those high in sugar or fat, dopamine levels rise, resulting in feelings of pleasure and reward, which can exacerbate cravings and promote overeating. Another neurotransmitter that regulates mood and appetite is serotonin, and disruptions in serotonin levels have been linked to increased cravings, particularly for carbohydrates, which can temporarily increase serotonin levels and improve mood.

3. **Brain Chemistry**: Cravings for specific foods are influenced by the brain's complex chemistry, which includes various regions and neurotransmitter systems. The reward pathway, which is centered on regions such as the nucleus accumbens and ventral tegmental area, reacts to pleasurable stimuli, including food, by releasing dopamine and reinforcing rewarding behaviors. When we have cravings, this reward pathway becomes hyperactive, resulting in increased motivation to seek out and consume highly rewarding foods. Furthermore, regions involved in decision-

making and impulse control, such as the prefrontal cortex, may be less active during cravings, making it more difficult to resist temptation and maintain self-control.

Overall, the physiological factors that influence cravings are complex and multifaceted, with intricate interactions between hormones, neurotransmitters, and brain chemistry. Understanding these biological mechanisms allows people to gain insight into the underlying causes of their cravings and develop effective management strategies, ultimately promoting healthier eating habits and overall well-being.

Types of cravings: emotional, physical, and habitual.

Cravings are classified into three types: emotional, physical, and habitual, each with its own set of triggers and characteristics.

1. **Emotional Cravings**: Emotional cravings stem from psychological factors rather than physical hunger. These cravings are often triggered by specific emotions or mood states, such as stress, sadness, boredom, loneliness, or anxiety. People may have a strong desire to eat certain foods as a means of comfort, distraction, or emotional relief. Emotional cravings are frequently associated with

comfort foods, which are highly palatable and typically high in calories and associated with positive emotions or memories. Examples include ice cream after a breakup, chocolate after a stressful day, and chips when bored.

2. **Physical Cravings**: These cravings are caused by the body's physiological needs, indicating nutrient or energy imbalances. Physical cravings, as opposed to emotional cravings, are usually more general and unrelated to specific emotional states. For example, craving salty foods could indicate a need for electrolytes, whereas craving protein-rich foods could indicate a need for amino acids. Physical cravings can also be caused by blood sugar

fluctuations or hormonal imbalance. It's critical to listen to your body and satisfy these cravings with nutritious foods that meet your nutritional requirements.

3. **Habitual Cravings**: Repeated behaviors and environmental cues can trigger conditioned responses and automatic cravings. Specific eating-related situations, contexts, or routines are frequently responsible for these cravings. For example, if you snack frequently while watching television or crave a sugary treat after dinner, these behaviors can become habitual, and cravings may arise automatically in those situations. Breaking habitual cravings entails identifying the cues or triggers that drive

the behavior and consciously replacing them with healthier options. New, healthier habits can be formed over time and with consistent effort.

Understanding the various types of cravings can help people identify their triggers and develop effective management strategies. Whether it's practicing mindfulness to address emotional cravings, nourishing the body with nutrient-dense foods to satisfy physical cravings, or reshaping routines to break habitual cravings, a holistic approach to cravings can benefit overall well-being and promote healthier eating habits.

Common myths about cravings

Misconceptions about cravings abound, frequently leading to misunderstandings about their nature, causes, and consequences. Dispelling these myths is critical for promoting a more accurate understanding of cravings and healthier ways to manage them. Here are some common misconceptions.

1. Cravings are entirely a matter of willpower: Cravings are often misunderstood as a sign of weakness or a lack of willpower. Cravings are complex phenomena influenced by a variety of biological, psychological, and environmental factors. While willpower is a factor in resisting cravings, it is not the only one; hormonal imbalances, neurotransmitter activity, and emotional triggers all contribute to cravings.

2. Cravings indicate a nutritional deficiency: While some cravings may reflect specific nutrient requirements (for example, craving red meat due to iron deficiency), the majority of cravings are not directly related to nutritional deficiencies. Cravings are frequently motivated by psychological or physiological factors, such as emotions, habits, or hormonal fluctuations. Cravings must be addressed holistically rather than assuming they are caused by a lack of nutrients.

3. Ignoring cravings will make them go away: Some people believe that ignoring or suppressing cravings will eventually cause them to vanish. Ignoring cravings,

on the other hand, can frequently have the opposite effect, increasing intensity or frequency over time. Cravings are signals from the body that something is out of balance, and it is critical to address the underlying causes rather than simply suppress them.

4. Cravings are always bad: While indulging in unhealthy cravings on a regular basis can have negative health consequences, occasional indulgences are normal and can even be beneficial to mental well-being. Complete self-denial can result in feelings of deprivation, which can fuel binge eating or disordered eating patterns.

When it comes to satisfying cravings, striking a balance and practicing moderation is critical.

5. Cravings are limited to people with poor diets: Cravings can affect anyone, regardless of their dietary habits or overall health status. While certain dietary patterns or nutrient deficiencies can affect the frequency or intensity of cravings, they are not limited to people who eat poorly. Cravings can be triggered by stress, emotions, hormonal fluctuations, and learned behaviors, regardless of diet quality.

6. Cravings are uncontrollable: Although cravings can feel overwhelming at times,

they can be managed and reduced in intensity using a variety of strategies. These may include identifying triggers, practicing mindfulness, developing healthier habits, addressing emotional needs, and providing the body with balanced meals. Individuals can gain greater control over their cravings and make more mindful food choices by becoming more aware and focused.

Part II: The Sneaky Method

Explaining the idea of the "sneaky Method": moving the emphasis from constraint to fulfillment

A paradigm shift in how we approach controlling cravings and accomplishing long-term weight loss is represented by the "sneaky method" concept. The "sneaky method" advocates for a more holistic and balanced approach that emphasizes fulfillment and satisfaction, as opposed to relying solely on restrictive diets and sheer willpower.

The premise behind the **"sneaky method"** is that traditional weight loss methods frequently emphasize restriction and deprivation, which can result in feelings of failure and frustration as well as rebound overeating. The "sneaky approach" proposes investigating alternate avenues to addressing cravings while concurrently promoting overall well-being, as opposed to continuously fighting against cravings and attempting to suppress them.

Suppose there were a front door and a back door on a house. The front door is a metaphor for the traditional weight loss strategy, which is marked by rigid calorie counting, restrictive diet plans, and complete food elimination. Although this strategy might help some people in the short run, eating satisfaction and enjoyment are frequently sacrificed in the process.

As an alternative, the "sneaky method" emphasizes understanding the underlying causes of cravings and coming up with novel, satisfying ways to satisfy those needs without turning to unhealthy habits.

Rather than merely prohibiting oneself from consuming sweets entirely, the "sneaky approach" suggests investigating the reasons behind one's cravings. Is it habitual, the result of stress, or something else entirely? People can then look for healthier ways to meet those needs after determining the underlying causes. This could be developing more nutrient-dense, filling foods that still satiate their sweet tooth in their diet, practicing mindfulness, or discovering alternate stress-relieving techniques.

Comparably, rather than rigorously following rules from outside sources, the "sneaky approach" promotes mindful eating and paying attention to one's body's signals of hunger and satiety. People can develop a healthier relationship with food and lose weight in a long-lasting way by emphasizing eating wholesome, satisfying foods and experiencing joy and pleasure when they eat.

In the end, adopting a more compassionate and balanced approach that puts fulfillment, enjoyment, and general well-being first replaces the idea that weight loss is a struggle of restriction and willpower. This is what the "Sneaky approach" concept ultimately represents. Opening the "sneaky approach" can help people find a new route that results in long-term success and a happier, healthier connection with food.

Why traditional diets don't work well at satisfying cravings

Conventional dieting frequently fails to effectively address cravings for a number of reasons:

1. **Emphasis on Restriction**: Strict guidelines and limitations are the hallmark of traditional diets, which frequently call for people to cut out entire food groups or significantly lower their caloric intake. This can cause severe cravings for foods that are off-limits, even though it might result in temporary weight loss. When cravings unavoidably occur, restriction can make one feel deprived and guilty or like a failure.

2. **Ignoring the Causes**: A lot of conventional diets neglect to address the

emotional triggers, stress, boredom, or hormonal fluctuations that are the root causes of cravings. These diets only concentrate on lowering calorie intake or eliminating particular foods, rather than investigating the reasons behind cravings. Long-term dietary changes can be difficult to stick with if the underlying causes of cravings are not addressed.

3. **Lack of Sustainability**: Conventional diets frequently advocate for quick fixes or rapid weight loss by putting excessive restrictions on calories or eating schedules. These methods seldom work over the long haul, even though they might produce some initial results. People may eventually become frustrated with the strict rules of

the diet and give up on it completely because they find it difficult to follow.

4. The "all-or-nothing" mentality is one that is frequently fostered by traditional diets, leading people to believe that they are either totally off track or closely following the diet's guidelines. When it comes to controlling cravings, this binary way of thinking can be harmful. People may experience guilt or shame when they eventually give in to cravings, which can result in a cycle of restriction and overindulgence, rather than learning how to manage cravings in a balanced way.

5. **Lack of Flexibility**: Conventional diets frequently have strict guidelines that don't

give much leeway for personal preferences, cravings, or lifestyle choices. It may be difficult for people to find a sustainable eating strategy that suits their particular requirements and tastes because of this lack of flexibility. Long-term dietary changes are hard to stick to without flexibility.

Generally, because they place more emphasis on restriction than on identifying and treating the underlying causes of cravings, traditional dieting techniques frequently fall short of providing effective relief. Adopting a more holistic approach that prioritizes balance, flexibility, and addressing the underlying causes of cravings is crucial for managing cravings and achieving sustainable weight loss

The sneaky method tenets of moderation, substitution, and mindfulness are introduced.

Traditional methods frequently leave us feeling stuck in a cycle of restriction and deprivation in our quest for effective craving management and sustainable weight loss. A welcome substitute, though, is provided by the principles of the sneaky approach—a comprehensive strategy that prioritizes long-term success, fulfillment, and balance.

1. **Mindfulness**: A practice that encourages us to develop awareness and presence in our eating habits, mindfulness is at the foundation of the sneaky approach principles. Being mindful helps us become more aware of the feelings and ideas that underlie our cravings as well as the signals our bodies give us when we are hungry or full. Slowing down and focusing on our eating experience can help us become more aware of our cravings and make more deliberate decisions about what and how much we eat.

2. **Substitution**: The sneaky approach suggests substituting healthier foods that still satiate our cravings rather than just forgoing the foods we simply cannot stand. Without sacrificing our health objectives, we can indulge in the tastes and textures we love by experimenting with inventive swaps and substitutions. Substitution enables us to satiate cravings in a more balanced and nourishing way. Examples of substitution include replacing sugary snacks with fruit, making homemade versions of our favorite treats, and experimenting with healthy substitutes.

3. **Moderation**: At the heart of the sneaky approach's tenets is the notion that, when

consumed in sensible amounts, every food can have a place in a balanced diet. Instead of categorizing foods as "good" or "bad," moderation inspires us to eat in a flexible and mindful manner. We can prevent feelings of deprivation and guilt while still moving closer to our health and weight loss objectives by allowing ourselves to enjoy a wide range of foods in moderation.

When combined, these Sneaky approach tenets offer a practical guide for controlling cravings and reaching long-term weight loss. Through the practice of mindfulness, substitution, and moderation, we can establish a more positive connection with food, overcome the pattern of restriction and deprivation, and find a more satisfying and well-rounded eating style.

Come along with us as we take the sneaky approach, a journey that promises greater happiness, fulfillment, and overall well-being in addition to physical transformation.

Case studies demonstrating the sneaky approach method's effective use

Case Study 1: Eating Consciously to Reduce Stress

During her hectic professional days, Esther frequently found herself reaching for unhealthy snacks. She discovered that stress eating was turning into a habit that was impeding her attempts to lose weight as she battled to control her cravings. Sarah made the conscious decision to change her eating habits after learning about the cunning strategy.

She began by dedicating a specific period of time each day to mindful eating. Sarah would stop and listen to her body for a few minutes before eating, noting any physical feelings of hunger or fullness. She made an effort to savor every bite of food during meals and snacks, focusing on its flavors, textures, and sensations.

Esther started to observe minor modifications in her eating patterns as she engaged in mindfulness exercises. She learned to distinguish between genuine hunger and emotional cravings as she grew more perceptive of her body's hunger cues. She discovered that by taking her time and enjoying her food, she was able to feel content with smaller servings and was no longer compelled to overindulge or mindlessly snack.

Esther eventually managed to escape the cycle of stress eating thanks to her mindful eating practice. She was able to lose weight and develop a more healthy relationship with food by addressing the underlying emotions that were causing her cravings and discovering more constructive ways to deal with stress.

Case Study 2: Using Healthy Substitutes Instead of

John, who called himself a "chocoholic," found it difficult to control his cravings for sweets, which frequently made it difficult for him to eat a balanced diet. John, who was determined to find a solution, made the decision to use the sneaky approach principle of substitution by looking for healthier substitutes for his favorite treats.

John tried creating his own chocolates at home with premium ingredients and natural sweeteners, as an alternative to grabbing store-bought chocolates that are packed with sugar and bad fats. He found recipes for nuts and dates that made for healthy energy balls, and for fruit covered in dark chocolate that was a satisfyingly sweet treat.

John discovered that he could still satiate his cravings while providing his body with nutritious ingredients by switching out his typical sugary snacks for healthier options. He stopped craving sugary treats as his taste buds became accustomed to the inherent sweetness of whole foods.

John was able to overcome his dependency on processed sugars and create a more well-rounded snacking strategy by using the substitution technique. He lost weight and experienced increased energy and general well-being by making tiny, gradual adjustments to his eating habits.

These case studies demonstrate how controlling cravings and achieving long-term weight loss are both possible goals when using the sneaky method approach. People can break free from restrictive dieting, cultivate healthier habits, and have a more satisfying relationship with food by adopting concepts like mindfulness,

substitution, and moderation into their
everyday lives.

Part 3: Mindfulness and Craving Awareness

Mindfulness is important for managing cravings.

Mindfulness is important in managing cravings because it raises awareness of the thoughts, emotions, and bodily sensations that contribute to them. Individuals who practice mindfulness can gain a better understanding of their cravings and learn to respond to them in a more intentional and empowered manner. Here are several major reasons why mindfulness is important in managing cravings:

1. **Increased Awareness**: Mindfulness is the practice of paying attention to the present moment without passing judgment. Mindfulness practice can help people become more aware of the triggers, patterns, and underlying emotions that lead to cravings. This increased awareness enables them to recognize cravings as they occur and understand the factors that contribute to them.

2. **Response Flexibility**: Mindfulness helps people become more flexible in how they respond to cravings. Rather than reacting impulsively or giving in to cravings, mindfulness allows people to pause, observe their cravings objectively, and choose a response that is consistent with their values and goals. This could mean finding alternative ways to meet underlying needs or simply allowing the craving to pass without acting on it.

3. **Emotional Regulation**: Cravings are frequently associated with emotions such as stress, anxiety, boredom, and sadness. Mindfulness practices, such as deep breathing, body scans, and meditation, can help people regulate their emotions and

reduce the intensity of cravings. Individuals who learn to sit with unpleasant emotions without seeking immediate relief through food can develop healthier coping mechanisms and reduce their reliance on emotional eating.

4. Increased Self-Compassion: Mindfulness promotes self-compassion and kindness, both of which are necessary for effective craving management. Rather than criticizing themselves for cravings or perceived "failures" in resisting them, people can practice self-compassion by acknowledging their humanity and responding to cravings with kindness and understanding. This compassionate approach reduces the guilt or shame associated with cravings and promotes a healthier relationship with food and oneself.

5. **Increased Sensory Awareness:**

Mindfulness entails tuning into the sensory experience of eating, such as the taste, texture, and aroma of food. Individuals who eat mindfully can derive more pleasure and satisfaction from their meals, reducing the likelihood of overeating or reaching for additional snacks to satisfy cravings. Paying attention to hunger and fullness cues can also help people distinguish between genuine hunger and cravings caused by other factors.

Overall, mindfulness is an effective tool for managing cravings because it increases awareness, promotes response flexibility, regulates emotions, fosters self-compassion, and enhances sensory awareness. Individuals who incorporate mindfulness practices into their daily lives can develop healthier eating habits, break the cycle of emotional eating, and achieve greater balance and well-being.

Three methods for cultivating mindfulness are self-reflection, journaling, and meditation.

Practicing mindfulness can increase your awareness of the present moment and yourself. Here are some methods to attempt:

1. **Meditation**: This is arguably the most widely used method of cultivating mindfulness. The practice of meditation involves bringing your mind back to the present moment when it strayed from your breathing, physical sensations, thoughts, or sounds. In addition to body scan meditation, other types of meditation include mindfulness meditation and loving-kindness meditation.

2. **Journaling**: Composing can be a highly useful mindfulness tool. You can write down your feelings, experiences, and thoughts in a daily journal. You can increase your awareness of your thoughts and emotions by engaging in this practice. To assist you in reflecting and developing a positive outlook, you can also utilize gratitude journals or journaling prompts.

3. **Self-reflection**: Being mindful requires taking the time to consider your past encounters, deeds, and feelings. It's possible to schedule time each day or week to think back on your feelings, your experiences, and your personal development. You can achieve this by journaling, spending time in quiet

reflection, or even just having a conversation with a therapist or close friend.

4. **Body Scan:** Body Scan is a mindfulness exercise where you systematically concentrate on various body parts, starting from your toes and working your way up to your head. Focusing on each body part, you can notice any sensations without passing judgment. Through this practice, you'll be able to recognize tense or uncomfortable spots on your body and increase your awareness of it.

5. **Mindful Walking**: Take up mindful walking as an alternative to hopping from

place to place. Become aware of every step you take, the feel of your feet hitting the ground, and your body's movements. You can enjoy the sights, sounds, and smells of your surroundings as you stroll. You can learn to be mindful and enjoy the little things in life, like walking, by practicing this.

6. **Mindful Eating:** When you eat, take the time to appreciate every taste and scent of the food. Observe your feelings before, during, and after meals. You can improve your relationship with food and increase your awareness of your body's hunger and fullness cues by practicing mindful eating.

7. **Gratitude Exercise**: Developing an attitude of gratitude is crucial to mindfulness. Whether it's a delicious meal, a gorgeous sunset, or a supportive friend, set aside some time each day to reflect on your blessings. You can either write down three things for which you are thankful each day, or you can just take a moment to be silently thankful.

Keep in mind that developing your mindfulness takes patience and practice. Perfectionism is not the goal; rather, it's about developing a more robust sense of presence in your day-to-day existence and approaching your experiences with a nonjudgmental awareness.

Identifying and comprehending craving triggers through mindfulness

Mindfulness allows you to identify and understand craving triggers by becoming aware of the thoughts, emotions, sensations, and situations that precede cravings. Here's how to use mindfulness to identify and comprehend your craving triggers:

1. **Mindful Observation**: Practice remaining fully present in the moment without passing judgment. When you have a craving, pay attention to what is going

on in your mind and body. Notice any thoughts, emotions, or physical sensations that arise without reacting.

2. **Body Awareness**: Pay attention to how your body responds to a craving. Take note of any tension, restlessness, or discomfort you may be feeling. Physical sensations can sometimes be used to predict when a craving will occur.

3. **Emotional Awareness**: Cravings are frequently associated with particular emotions such as stress, boredom, loneliness, or sadness. Practice identifying and labeling your emotions as they arise during the day. Take note of any patterns

or triggers that appear to be related to cravings.

4. **Thought Patterns**: Recognize the thoughts and beliefs that accompany your cravings. Observe any recurring thoughts or stories you tell yourself about why you need to indulge in the craving. Recognize that these are just thoughts, and you have the ability to choose how to respond to them.

5. **Mindful Eating**: Be aware of your eating habits and the circumstances that surround your food cravings. Consider whether you eat in response to certain triggers, such as watching TV, being stressed, or being around certain people.

Mindful eating can help you become more conscious of your eating habits and make better choices.

6. **Mindful Pause**: Rather than giving in to a craving right away, try taking a mindful pause. Take a moment to observe your thoughts, emotions, and sensations without judgment. Consider if giving in to the craving is consistent with your values and long-term goals.

7. **Mindfulness Practices**: Practice mindfulness regularly, such as meditation, deep breathing exercises, or yoga. These exercises can help you improve your self-awareness and self-regulation, making it

easier to identify and manage craving triggers.

By identifying and comprehending your craving triggers through the practice of mindfulness, you can cultivate more constructive coping mechanisms and make more deliberate choices regarding your response to cravings in a manner that aligns with your personal objectives and values.

Practical exercises for increasing craving awareness

Practicing exercises to increase craving awareness can help you become more aware of your triggers and reactions, allowing you to develop healthier responses. Here are some practical exercises that you can try.

1. **Craving Journal:** Keep a journal in which you record your cravings throughout the day. Whenever you have a craving, write down the time of day, the trigger (e.g., emotion, situation), the type of craving (e.g., food, substance), and the intensity of the craving. Take note of any

patterns or common triggers that emerge over time.

2. **Mindful Eating**: Set aside a few minutes to practice mindful eating with a small serving of your favorite dish. Before taking a bite, use all of your senses to notice the food's color, texture, smell, and any mouth sensations. Take a small bite and chew slowly, paying attention to the flavor and texture of the food. Take note of any thoughts or emotions that arise while you are eating. This exercise can help you become more conscious of your eating habits and how cravings manifest.

3. **STOP Technique**: When you notice a craving arising, pause for a moment and use the STOP technique.
- S: Immediately stop what you are doing.
- T: To center yourself, take a few deep breaths.
- O: Observe your thoughts, emotions, and physical sensations without judgment.
- P: Maintain awareness and choose how you want to respond to the craving mindfully.

4. **Urge Surfing**: Imagine your craving as a wave, with the peak representing your strongest desire to indulge. Sit back and concentrate on your breath. As the craving wave builds, observe your body's sensations and thoughts without resisting

or acting on them. Notice how the intensity of the craving varies over time, eventually subsiding like a wave returning to the ocean. This exercise can help you overcome cravings without giving in to them impulsively.

5. **Body Scan Meditation**: Use a body scan meditation to develop awareness of the physical sensations associated with cravings. Lie down or sit comfortably and direct your attention to each part of your body, beginning with your toes and progressing to your head. As you scan each body part, note any areas of tension, discomfort, or sensation. Pay special attention to any sensations that arise during cravings.

6. **Labeling Thoughts and Emotions**: Practice labeling your thoughts and emotions as they occur throughout the day. When you notice a craving or the thoughts and emotions that accompany it, mentally label them as "craving," "desire," "anxiety," "stress," and so on. This simple act of labeling can help you distance yourself from your thoughts and emotions, allowing you to observe them more objectively.

7. **Gratitude Practice**: Use gratitude to shift your focus away from cravings. Take a few moments every day to reflect on three things you're grateful for. This practice can help you develop a more

positive mindset and reduce craving intensity by focusing on what you already have rather than what you want.

Consistent practice of these exercises can help you become more aware of your cravings, understand their underlying causes, and develop healthier coping strategies to effectively manage them.

Part IV: Strategies for Substitution

An introduction to using substitution to control cravings

Strong impulses to indulge in food, drugs, or behaviors—such as eating—are known as cravings. Though it's normal to occasionally feel cravings, if they're ignored, they may occasionally result in bad decisions or actions. Substitution is an efficient way to control cravings.

Substitution is putting an unhealthy substitute for the item you're craving in place of it while still satisfying the same underlying need or want. Cravings can be lessened and decisions that support your values and objectives can be made by shifting your attention to a more constructive or positive option.

This is the process of substitution:

1. **Recognize the Craving**: Understanding what and why you are craving something is the first step towards using substitution to control cravings. Is it a compulsive phone-checking habit, a craving for a particular food, or a substance like nicotine or caffeine? For a moment, accept the craving without passing judgment.

2. **Recognize the Need**: Next, make an effort to determine what need or desire lies at the root of the craving. Emotional or physical cues like stress, boredom, loneliness, or hunger can trigger cravings. You can select a replacement that more successfully satisfies the craving by determining its underlying cause.

3. **Pick a Healthier Substitute**: After determining the craving's underlying need, pick a healthier substitute to meet it. For instance, instead of reaching for a candy bar when you're craving something sweet, try reaching for a piece of fruit. Try chewing gum or going for a quick walk if you're craving a cigarette to boost your energy and relieve stress.

4. **Exercise Mindfulness**: As you replace your cravings with healthier options, exercise mindfulness by observing your body's and mind's reactions. After making the switch, observe any alterations in your energy levels, mood, or cravings. You can find the substitutions that work best for you and adjust as necessary if you are present and pay attention.

5. **Develop Healthy Habits**: You can develop new, health-promoting habits over time by regularly replacing your cravings with healthier options. You'll learn more constructive ways to deal with stress and cravings rather than falling back on unhealthy coping strategies.

It's crucial to keep in mind that controlling cravings requires patience and persistence, as it takes time to get used to. As you try out various substitutions and figure out what suits you the best, be kind to yourself. It's okay to give in to a craving if you make a mistake. Instead, make the most of it as a chance to consider what set off the craving and how you might react differently the next time.

You can take proactive measures to make healthier decisions and foster greater well-being in your life by adding substitution to your toolkit for managing cravings.

Sugar, salt, and fat are healthy substitutes for common craving triggers.

Making wholesome decisions while satisfying your cravings can be achieved by looking for healthy substitutes for typical craving triggers like fat, sugar, and salt. These are a few choices:

1. **Sugar Cravings**: - Fresh Fruit: Naturally sweet fruits such as bananas, apples, berries, and oranges can satiate

your sweet tooth and provide you with fiber, vitamins, and minerals.

Snack on Dried Fruit: If you're looking for a concentrated sweetness without added sugars, try dates, figs, apricots, or raisins.

The leaves of the Stevia rebaudiana plant are used to make stevia, a naturally occurring sweetener that has no calories. It can be added to recipes for baked goods, beverages, and other applications in place of sugar.

Choose Dark Chocolate: Dark chocolate with a high cocoa content (at least 70%) is better for you than milk chocolate because it has more health benefits and less sugar.

2. **Cravings for Salt**: - Herbs and Spices: Aim to flavor your food with herbs and spices rather than salt. Try adding different spices to your food, such as garlic, ginger, cumin, paprika, basil, cilantro, and rosemary, to give them more flavor and complexity.

- **Sea Vegetables: To** add flavor and natural sodium to soups, salads, or stir-fries, add sea vegetables like nori, dulse, or kombu.

- **Citrus Juice:** Without using salt, squeeze fresh lemon or lime juice over salads, seafood, or vegetables to add brightness and acidity.

Almonds, walnuts, pumpkin seeds, and sunflower seeds are a few examples of unsalted nuts and seeds that make a satisfying crunch and a good source of healthy fats.

3. **Cravings for Fat:** - Avocado: If you're craving creamy, heart-healthy monounsaturated fats, spread mashed avocado on toast, add slices to salads or sandwiches, or blend it into smoothies.
- **Nuts and Nut Butters**: For satisfying protein and fats, eat a tablespoon of nut butter or a handful of nuts as a snack. You can also add nuts to smoothies, oats, and yogurt.
Greek yogurt: Go for the plain, unsweetened variety; it's high in probiotics and protein. For extra taste, sprinkle some almonds, fresh fruit, or honey on top.

Extra virgin olive oil is a healthy fat source that can be used for cooking, drizzling salads, or dipping bread. To get the most flavor and nutritional value, choose cold-pressed, premium olive oil.

Your body will receive the necessary nutrients and you will be able to satiate your cravings for sugar, salt, and fat while also improving your general health and well-being.

Creating enticing and wholesome replacement meals and snacks

It takes imagination and a commitment to using complete, nutrient-dense foods to create filling and healthy substitute meals and snacks. Here are some mouthwatering substitutes for typical cravings:

1. **Sweet Tooth Substitutes:** - Greek Yogurt Parfait: combine plain Greek yogurt with chopped nuts or granola, fresh berries, and a drizzle of honey or maple syrup to create a creamy, filling dessert.
- **Frozen Banana "Ice Cream":** Blend frozen bananas until creamy, adding a small amount of milk or plant-based milk if desired. For added flavor, incorporate flavorings such as nut butter, vanilla extract, or cocoa powder.

- **Chia Seed Pudding:** Blend together chia seeds, milk, and sweetener (such as maple syrup or agave nectar) and refrigerate until the mixture thickens into a pudding-like consistency. For extra taste and texture, sprinkle nuts, coconut flakes, or fruits on top.

- **Roasted Chickpeas:** Combine cooked chickpeas with your preferred seasonings (such as cumin, paprika, or garlic powder) and bake until crispy. This is an alternative to salty snacks. Enjoy as a high-protein, crunchy snack.

- Homemade Popcorn: For a flavorful and filling snack, season air-popped popcorn or plain popcorn with a small amount of olive oil, nutritional yeast, sea salt, and a few herbs.

Vegetables such as sweet potatoes, beets, or zucchini can be thinly sliced, tossed with olive oil and seasonings, and baked until crispy. This recipe makes about 8 servings. Savor this wholesome take on store-bought chips.

3. **Options for Healthy Fats**: - Avocado Toast: For a filling and wholesome snack or dinner, spread mashed avocado on whole-grain toast and garnish with sliced tomatoes, feta cheese, and a drizzle of balsamic glaze.

A nutrient-dense take on traditional sushi rolls is the Salmon and Avocado Sushi Roll, which is made of cooked quinoa, sliced avocado, cucumber, and cooked salmon rolled in nori seaweed sheets.

- **Nutty Quinoa Salad:** Toss cooked quinoa with diced avocado, chopped bell peppers, cucumbers, and toasted nuts (almonds, walnuts) in a lemon-tahini dressing to create a tasty and substantial salad.

4. **Nourishment and Hydration**:

- Infused Water: To add taste and hydration, infuse plain water with fresh fruits (like lemon, cucumber, berries), herbs (like mint, basil), or cucumber slices.

Make your own smoothies at home: Blend your preferred fruits, leafy greens, Greek yogurt or protein powder, and a liquid (such as water, almond milk, or coconut water) to create a wholesome and revitalizing snack or meal substitute.

While enjoying these healthy meal and snack options, keep in mind to pay attention to portion control and pay attention to your body's signals of hunger and fullness. You can satiate your cravings, nourish your body, and advance general health and well-being by including a range of whole, nutrient-dense foods in your diet.

Adding diversity and originality to replacement tactics

Sustainable and enjoyable healthy eating can be achieved by incorporating creativity and variety into substitution strategies. The following advice can help you infuse your substitution strategy with more originality and variety:

1:Examine Various Tastes and Textures: To give your meals taste and excitement, try a variety of herbs, spices, sauces, and condiments. To improve the flavor of your food, try adding components like pesto, miso paste, sriracha, or curry powder.

2. **Blend and Blend Ingredients**:

Experiment with different combinations of ingredients to create original flavor combinations. For instance, in a stir-fry or salad, combine savory components like grilled chicken or tofu with sweet fruits like pineapple or mango.

3. **Get Inspired by Global Cuisines**: To

add some spice to your meals, consider getting ideas from different cuisines around the globe. Investigate recipes from Middle Eastern, Asian, Mexican, or Mediterranean cuisines, and make substitutions using their customary ingredients and cooking methods.

Play with Colors and Presentation: Use a range of colorful fruits, vegetables, grains, and proteins to create meals that are aesthetically pleasing. To add visual interest to your dishes, try experimenting with different textures and shapes. Add some flair to your meals by garnishing them with toasted nuts, citrus zest, or fresh herbs.

5. Explore New Cooking Techniques: Broaden your culinary horizons by experimenting with various cooking techniques, including grilling, roasting, steaming, sautéing, and slow cooking. Every technique gives ingredients a distinct flavor and texture, enabling you to make a variety of mouthwatering dishes.

6. **Recreate Your Favorite Comfort Foods:** Use your imagination in the kitchen to create a healthier version of your go-to comfort foods. For instance, instead of using regular dough to make pizza crust, use spiralized vegetables instead of pasta, or replace fried chicken with baked or grilled chicken tenders.

7. **Try New Ingredients**: Instead of relying solely on traditional staples like rice, pasta, and flour, consider trying new ingredients like quinoa, cauliflower rice, lentil pasta, or almond flour. These substitutes can give your meals more diversity and offer varying nutritional profiles.

8. Involve Friends and Family: By preparing meals together, you can make mealtimes a creative and social occasion. To keep things fresh and motivating, share recipes, confer on culinary techniques, and work together on meal concepts.

9. Maintain a Recipe Journal: List your go-to substitute recipes and dinner suggestions in an electronic recipe book or folder. This enables you to experiment with new versions over time and return to and adjust recipes according to your preferences.

10. Have an open mind and be curious: In your culinary explorations, adopt an attitude of openness and curiosity. Be open to experimenting with different flavors, foods, and cooking methods, and don't give up if an experiment doesn't work out the first time. It's enjoyable to learn from your mistakes!

You can make long-term sustainable healthy eating enjoyable, flavorful, and creative by adding diversity and creativity into your substitution strategies. Continue experimenting, investigating, and learning new approaches to satisfying your palate and nourishing your body!

Part V: Moderation and Balance

The function of moderation in long-term weight management

Moderation is essential for long-term weight management because it encourages sustainable and balanced eating habits. Here is why moderation is important:

1. **Balanced Nutrition**: Moderation allows you to eat a wide range of foods while still meeting your nutritional requirements. Incorporate a variety of fruits, vegetables, whole grains, lean proteins, and healthy fats into your diet in moderation to ensure that your body receives the nutrients it requires for optimal health and well-being.

2. **Flexible Eating**: Taking a moderate approach to eating allows for greater flexibility and enjoyment in your food choices. Rather than adhering to strict diets or eliminating entire food groups, you can incorporate your favorite foods in moderation, making it easier to stick to your eating plan over time.

3. Overeating Prevention: Moderation promotes mindful eating habits, which help to prevent overeating. When you allow yourself to eat small portions of your favorite foods without restriction, you are less likely to feel deprived and more likely to respond to your body's hunger and fullness cues.

4. Weight Maintenance: Moderation is essential for sustaining a healthy weight over time. Consuming foods in moderation and being mindful of portion sizes can help you manage your calorie intake and avoid excessive weight gain or loss.

5. **Psychological Well-Being:** Strict diets or extreme eating habits can cause feelings of deprivation, guilt, and frustration, which can ultimately undermine your weight loss efforts. Moderation fosters a healthy relationship with food by allowing for occasional indulgences without causing negative emotions or outcomes.

6. **Lifestyle Sustainability**: For long-term weight management, you must adopt eating habits that you can stick to. Moderation encourages a realistic and sustainable approach to eating, which makes it easier to maintain healthy habits over time.

7. **Health Benefits:** According to research, a balanced diet that includes a variety of foods in moderation is linked to a number of health benefits, including a lower risk of chronic diseases like heart disease, diabetes, and certain cancers.

8. **Food Enjoyment:** Food is more than just a source of energy for the body; it also provides pleasure and enjoyment. Moderation allows you to savor and appreciate your meals without feeling guilty or deprived, fostering a positive relationship with food and improving overall health.

To summarize, moderation is critical for long-term weight management because it promotes balanced nutrition, prevents overeating, promotes psychological well-being, and encourages sustainable lifestyle habits. By eating in moderation, you can achieve and maintain a healthy weight while still enjoying the foods you enjoy.

Strategies for maintaining moderation without deprivation

Moderation without deprivation entails taking a balanced approach to eating that allows you to enjoy your favorite foods while also maintaining a healthy lifestyle.

Here are some strategies to help you practice moderation more effectively:

1. **Mindful Eating:** Pay attention to your body's hunger and fullness cues and eat slowly so you can fully savor and enjoy your meal.

Avoid using electronic devices or watching television while eating, as these activities can encourage mindless eating.

2. **Portion Control**: Be aware of your portion sizes and aim to fill your plate with a variety of nutritious foods such as fruits, vegetables, lean proteins, and whole grains. Use smaller plates, bowls, and utensils to help you control portion sizes and avoid overeating.

3. **Plan Ahead**: Plan your meals and snacks ahead of time to ensure that you always have nutritious options on hand. Incorporate a variety of foods that you enjoy into your meal plan, and allow yourself to indulge in small amounts of your favorite treats on occasion.

4. **Follow the 80/20 Rule**: Aim to make healthy choices about 80% of the time, while allowing yourself to indulge in less nutritious foods the other 20% of time. This approach promotes flexibility and enjoyment while also improving overall health and well-being.

5. **Satiate Cravings Mindfully**: When you have a craving for a certain food,

allow yourself to eat it in moderation without guilt. Savor the food's flavor and texture, and try not to overeat.

6. **Prioritize Quality Over Quantity:** Rather than depriving yourself of your favorite foods, opt for smaller portions of high-quality, nutrient-dense alternatives. Select a small piece of dark chocolate with a high cocoa content over a larger portion of milk chocolate.

7. **Practice Self-Compassion**: Be kind to yourself and avoid categorizing foods as "good" or "bad." Remember that all foods can be consumed in moderation as part of a balanced diet, and it is acceptable to indulge on occasion without judgment.

8. **Stay Active**: Incorporate regular physical activity into your daily routine to balance out occasional indulgences and promote overall health and well-being. Exercise can also help regulate appetite and improve mood, making it easier to maintain moderation in your eating habits.

9. **Keep a Food Journal:** Keeping track of your food intake and eating habits in a journal or app can help you stay accountable and identify patterns of overeating or emotional eating. Use the journal to evaluate your choices and make changes as needed.

10. **Seek Support**: Surround yourself with supportive friends, family members, or a registered dietitian who can offer encouragement, accountability, and guidance as you strive for moderation without deprivation.

By incorporating these strategies into your daily routine, you can develop a balanced eating style that allows you to enjoy your favorite foods while also supporting your health and well-being. Remember that moderation is about striking a sustainable balance that allows you to live life to the fullest.

Creating balanced meals and snacks to avoid excessive cravings

Balanced meals and snacks are essential for avoiding extreme cravings and maintaining consistent energy levels

throughout the day. Here's how to prepare balanced meals and snacks:

1. **Incorporate Protein:** Make sure to include protein in every meal and snack. Protein keeps you feeling full and satisfied, lowering the likelihood of cravings. Protein-rich foods include lean meats, poultry, fish, eggs, tofu, tempeh, beans, lentils, Greek yogurt, cottage cheese, and nuts.

2. **Consume Fiber-Rich Foods**: Fiber regulates blood sugar levels and promotes feelings of fullness. To increase your fiber intake, include plenty of fruits, vegetables, whole grains, legumes, nuts, and seeds in your meals and snacks.

3. **Include Healthy Fats**: Healthy fats aid in satiety and nutrient absorption. Incorporate healthy fats into your meals and snacks from avocado, nuts, seeds, olive oil, fatty fish (such as salmon and sardines), and coconut products.

4. **Choose Complex Carbohydrates:** Choose complex carbohydrates that are high in fiber and nutrients over refined carbohydrates, which can cause blood sugar spikes and crashes. Complex carbohydrates include whole grains (such as brown rice, quinoa, oats, and barley), starchy vegetables (such as sweet potatoes and winter squash), and legumes.

5. **Macronutrient Balance**: Make sure each meal and snack contains a balanced amount of carbohydrates, protein, and fat. This helps to provide long-lasting energy and prevent cravings by maintaining stable blood sugar levels.

6. **Mindful Portioning**: Pay attention to portion sizes to avoid overeating and ensure you're getting the right nutrients. Use visual cues, such as the size of your palm or a deck of cards, to determine appropriate portion sizes for protein, grains, and fats.

7. **Stay Hydrated**: Drink plenty of water throughout the day to maintain hydration. Feelings of hunger can be symptoms of

dehydration. Drink plenty of water and incorporate hydrating foods like fruits and vegetables into your daily meals and snacks.

8. **Plan Ahead:** Set aside time to prepare balanced meals and snacks. This helps to ensure that you have nutritious options on hand when hunger strikes, lowering the likelihood of reaching for unhealthy, high-calorie foods.

9. **Listen to Your Body:** Pay attention to your body's hunger and fullness cues, and eat when you're hungry rather than when you're ravenous. Similarly, rather than eating until you're completely full, stop eating when you're comfortably satisfied.

10. **Include Variety:** To ensure that you're getting a diverse range of nutrients, incorporate a variety of foods into your meals and snacks. Experiment with different flavors, textures, and cuisines to keep your meals interesting and fulfilling.

You can avoid extreme cravings, maintain stable energy levels, and support overall health and well-being by preparing balanced meals and snacks that include a variety of protein, fiber, healthy fats, and complex carbohydrates.

Overcoming the guilt and shame associated with indulgence.

Overcoming the guilt and shame associated with indulgence is an important step toward developing a healthy relationship with food and promoting overall well-being. Here are some techniques to assist you in overcoming these negative emotions:

1. **Practice Self-Compassion**: Be kind and compassionate to yourself, particularly when it comes to food choices. Understand that it is normal and natural to indulge in treats on occasion,

and refrain from harsh self-criticism or judgment.

2. Challenge All-or-Nothing Thinking: Avoid thinking about food in black-and-white terms, labeling certain foods as "good" or "bad." Instead, adopt a more adaptable mindset that encourages moderation and balance. Recognize that a single indulgence does not define your entire eating habits or health.

3. Prioritize Balance and Moderation: Adopt a balanced eating strategy that includes a variety of foods in moderation. Allow yourself to eat indulgent foods on occasion without guilt, while also prioritizing nutrient-dense foods that nourish your body and promote your health.

4. **Reframe Negative Thoughts**: Examine your negative thoughts and beliefs about food and indulgence. Instead of seeing indulgence as a failure or weakness, consider it a normal and enjoyable part of life. Concentrate on the positive aspects of your experience, such as pleasure, enjoyment, and social connection.

5. **Practice Mindful Eating**: Develop mindfulness around eating by focusing on the sensory experience of food, such as taste, texture, and aroma. Eat slowly, savoring every bite, and pay attention to your body's hunger and fullness cues.

Mindful eating can help you establish a more positive and nonjudgmental relationship with food.

6. **Keep Emotions Separate from Food**: Avoid using food to deal with stress, boredom, or sadness. Instead, find other ways to manage your emotions, such as practicing relaxation techniques, participating in hobbies, or seeking help from friends or a therapist.

7. **Practice Gratitude**: Rather than dwelling on feelings of guilt or shame, express gratitude for the nourishing and enjoyable aspects of food. Appreciate the pleasure and satisfaction that indulgent foods can provide, and express gratitude

for the variety of food options available to you.

8. **Forgive Yourself**: If you overindulge or make decisions you later regret, practice self-forgiveness. Accept that everyone makes mistakes and release any feelings of guilt or shame. Instead of dwelling on the past, use the experience as an opportunity to learn and grow.

9. **Seek Support**: If you're feeling guilty or ashamed about food, seek help from friends, family members, or a therapist. Discussing your feelings with others can help you gain perspective, receive encouragement, and feel less alone in your struggles.

10. **Prioritize Health and Well-Being**: Instead of focusing on weight and appearance goals, prioritize your overall health and well-being. Participate in activities that nourish your body, mind, and spirit, such as regular physical activity, enough sleep, and meaningful social connections.

Implementing these strategies will help you overcome feelings of guilt and shame associated with indulging, develop a healthier relationship with food, and cultivate a more positive and balanced approach to eating and well-being.

Part VI: Conquering Particular Wants

Handling sugar and sweet tooth cravings

Although satisfying your cravings for sugar and sweets can be difficult, you can lessen their frequency and intensity by using the appropriate tactics. Here are some pointers to help you effectively control your cravings for sugar:

Consume Often, Balanced Meals: Missing meals or fasting for extended periods of time can cause blood sugar swings, which can set off cravings for sweets. To help control blood sugar levels and avoid cravings, try to eat balanced meals that include plenty of fruits and vegetables, fiber-rich carbohydrates, healthy fats, and protein.

Incorporate Protein and Good Fats: These foods can make you feel satiated and full, which lowers the chance that you'll have sugar cravings. Add lean meats, poultry, fish, eggs, tofu, beans, and nuts to your meals and snacks as protein sources. Include healthy fats as well, such as those found in avocados, nuts, seeds, olive oil, and fatty fish.

3. **Go for Whole Foods:** In place of heavily processed and refined foods, choose whole, minimally processed foods. Whole foods with natural sugars and fiber, such as fruits, vegetables, whole grains, legumes, and lean proteins, can help satiate your sweet tooth while supplying vital nutrients and encouraging fullness.

4. **Maintain Hydration**: Sometimes hunger or a sugar craving can be mistaken for dehydration. Stay hydrated and less

likely to experience false hunger cues by drinking lots of water throughout the day.

5. **Control Stress**: Stress can lead to cravings for sugary foods, which people often turn to when they're feeling down. Use stress-reduction methods to control your stress levels and lessen cravings, such as deep breathing, yoga, meditation, and spending time in nature.

6. **Get Appropriate Sleep:** Sleep deprivation can mess with hormones that regulate hunger and make you crave more sugary foods. To enhance general health and lessen cravings for sugar, aim for seven to nine hours of good sleep each night.

7. **Determine Triggers**: Observe the events, feelings, or pursuits that set off your desire for sugar. After you've determined what your triggers are, create alternate coping mechanisms to deal with them. Some ideas include taking a walk, meditating, or taking up a hobby.

8. **Reduce Temptation**: Make healthier food choices and keep sugary foods hidden from view to reduce your exposure to them. Store wholesome options such as fruits, vegetables, nuts, seeds, and whole-grain snacks in your fridge and pantry.

9. **Exercise Moderation**: Don't feel bad about indulging in moderation from time

to time in tiny servings of your favorite sweets. Complete self-deprivation may result in feelings of guilt and, in the end, may lead to overindulgence.

10. **Seek Support:** You might want to consult a registered dietitian, therapist, or support group if you're finding it difficult to control your sugar cravings on your own. They can support you in overcoming cravings and forming better eating habits by offering you individualized advice, accountability, and encouragement.

You can develop a balanced eating style that promotes your general health and well-being and lessen your cravings for sugar and sweets by putting these strategies into practice. Remind yourself that change takes time, so be kind to yourself and acknowledge your accomplishments as you go.

Controlling the need for savory and salty foods

Combining techniques to address the psychological and physiological aspects of cravings for savory and salty foods is necessary to manage them. These pointers will assist you in effectively controlling your cravings for savory and salty foods:

1. **Select Nutrient-Dense Alternatives:** Choose nutrient-dense snacks that fulfill your cravings and supply vital nutrients rather than processed salty snacks like pretzels or chips. Some of the examples are whole-grain crackers topped with cheese, roasted chickpeas, air-popped popcorn, and veggie sticks with hummus.

2. Use Tasty Herbs and Spices: Instead of relying too much on salt, use herbs and spices to make your food taste better. Try experimenting with different seasonings to give your dishes more depth and complexity, like garlic, onion powder, cumin, paprika, turmeric, basil, oregano, and thyme.

3. Eat More Foods High in Protein: Protein increases feelings of fullness and lessens the desire for savory and salty foods. Eat a diet high in protein to help stifle cravings and prolong feelings of fullness. Examples of such foods include lean meats, poultry, fish, eggs, tofu, tempeh, beans, and lentils.

4. Choose Healthy Fats: By giving your food more depth and flavor, healthy fats can help you eat less salt. To satiate your cravings for savory foods, include sources of healthy fats in your diet, such as avocado, nuts, seeds, olive oil, fatty fish, and coconut products.

5. Drink Plenty of Water: Occasionally, cravings for salty foods may indicate a dehydration state. To stay hydrated and lessen cravings, sip lots of water throughout the day. In addition to plain water, herbal teas and flavored sparkling water can be refreshing substitutes.

6. Mindful Eating: Be aware of your body's signals of hunger and fullness, and eat with awareness to prevent overindulging in salty foods. Enjoy the tastes and textures of your food as you eat it slowly, and stop eating when you're content but not too full.

7. **Restrict Your Consumption of Processed Foods**: Packaged snacks, frozen dinners, and canned soups are examples of processed foods that are high in sodium. To cut back on salt overall, limit these foods in your diet and opt for whole, minimally processed foods whenever possible.

8. **Plan Balanced Meals**: To help avoid cravings for particular food types, plan balanced meals that include a range of

flavors, textures, and nutrients. To increase satiety and satisfaction, try to incorporate a variety of fiber-rich foods, protein, healthy fats, and carbs in each meal.

9. **Manage Your Stress**: Dealing with negative emotions can lead to cravings for savory and salty foods, which can be triggered by stress. Use stress-reduction methods to control your stress levels and lessen cravings, such as deep breathing, yoga, meditation, and spending time in nature.

10. **Seek Support**: You might want to consult a registered dietitian or therapist if you're finding it difficult to control your

cravings for savory and salty foods. They can offer you strategies to beat cravings and form better eating habits, as well as individualized guidance and accountability.

You can develop a balanced eating style that promotes your general health and well-being and effectively control your cravings for savory and salty foods by putting these strategies into practice. Always remember to treat yourself with patience and acknowledge your accomplishments as you go.

Techniques for overcoming cravings for fatty foods

Although satisfying cravings for high-fat foods can be difficult, there are a few techniques you can employ to help control your cravings. The following advice is provided:

1. **Select Healthy Fats**: Use sources of healthy fats in your meals and snacks to help you satiate your cravings while also providing you with nutrition. Avocados, nuts, seeds, olive oil, avocado products, fatty fish (like salmon and mackerel), and coconut products are a few examples. In addition to offering you important fatty acids, these foods can make you feel full and content.

2. **Select Whole Foods**: Stay away from highly processed, high-fat options and instead go for whole, minimally processed foods. Because they include natural fats in

addition to other vital nutrients, whole foods such as fruits, vegetables, whole grains, lean proteins, and legumes are a healthier option when it comes to satisfying your cravings.

3. **Use Portion Control**: Rather than overindulging in high-fat foods when you're craving them, try to enjoy them in moderation. To encourage fullness and avoid overindulging, watch portion sizes and make sure your meals and snacks have a good ratio of fats, proteins, and carbohydrates.

4. **Eat More Fiber**: Eating more fiber-rich foods can make you feel full and content and lessen your desire for foods high in

fat. To boost your intake of fiber and support digestive health, include an abundance of fruits, vegetables, whole grains, legumes, nuts, and seeds in your diet.

5. **Drink Plenty of Water**: Occasionally, cravings for fatty foods may indicate a dehydration state. To stay hydrated and lessen cravings, sip lots of water throughout the day. In addition to plain water, herbal teas and flavored sparkling water can be refreshing substitutes.

6. **Eat Mindfully**: Be aware of your body's signals of hunger and fullness, and mindfully eat to prevent consuming excessive amounts of high-fat foods.

Enjoy the tastes and textures of your food as you eat it slowly, and stop eating when you're content but not too full.

7. **Recognize Triggers**: Keep an eye out for the circumstances, feelings, or pursuits that set off your desire for high-fat foods. After you've determined what your triggers are, create alternate coping mechanisms to deal with them. Some ideas include taking a walk, meditating, or taking up a hobby.

8. **Find Healthier Substitutes**: Seek for less-fattening substitutes for your preferred high-fat foods that will still satiate your cravings. Try baked kale chips or air-popped popcorn seasoned with

herbs and spices, for instance, if you're craving potato chips. Try out a variety of recipes and cooking techniques to find wholesome choices you enjoy.

9. **Manage Your Stress:** Stress can lead to cravings for foods heavy in fat because people use them as a coping mechanism for uncomfortable feelings. Use stress-reduction methods to control your stress levels and lessen cravings, such as deep breathing, yoga, meditation, and spending time in nature.

10. **Seek Support**: You might want to consult a registered dietitian or therapist if you're finding it difficult to control your cravings for high-fat foods on your own.

They can offer you strategies to beat cravings and form better eating habits, as well as individualized guidance and accountability.

You can develop a balanced eating style that promotes your general health and well-being and effectively control cravings for high-fat foods by putting these strategies into practice. Always remember to treat yourself with patience and acknowledge your accomplishments as you go.

Taking care of desires brought on by boredom or emotional tension

Creating alternate coping mechanisms to address underlying emotions and lessen the impulse to reach for food is necessary when managing cravings brought on by emotional stress or boredom. Here are some methods to help you control cravings brought on by boredom or emotional stress:

1. **Identify Triggers**: Be mindful of the feelings, circumstances, or activities that set off your hunger pangs. Maintain a journal to record your cravings and identify any trends or recurring triggers. You can create more focused strategies to deal with your triggers by identifying what they are.

2. **Engage in Mindfulness Practice**: To become more conscious of your thoughts, emotions, and physical sensations in the present, practice mindfulness. Take a moment to check in with yourself when you are experiencing cravings. Be mindful of any feelings or pressures that might be fueling the craving without passing judgment.

3. **Find Other Coping Strategies**: To deal with emotional stress or boredom, consider other coping mechanisms other than eating for solace or diversion. Exercises like deep breathing, yoga, meditation, journaling, music listening,

taking up a hobby, or taking a stroll in the outdoors are a few examples.

4. **Take Proactive Action to Address Emotional Needs**: Rather than using food as a coping mechanism for uncomfortable emotions, address underlying emotional needs. Seek professional counseling or therapy, connect with encouraging friends or family, engage in self-care activities that support your emotional health.

5. **Keep Moving**: Frequent movement helps improve mood, lower stress levels, and divert attention from cravings. Try to fit in some fun physical activities to your routine, like yoga, walking, jogging, dancing, or cycling. Stress can be reduced

and cravings can be lessened with even brief active intervals.

6. **Establish a Supportive Environment**: Surround yourself with individuals who are encouraging and establish an atmosphere that encourages healthy behaviors. Talk to friends or family who can support and hold you accountable about your objectives and difficulties. Reduce your exposure to unhealthy temptations and keep wholesome foods easily accessible in your home.

7. **Practice Self-Compassion**: When you are dealing with challenging emotions or cravings, especially, treat yourself with kindness and compassion. Recognize that

cravings are common and try not to be judgmental or critical of yourself. As you would a friend in a comparable circumstance, show yourself compassion and understanding.

8. **Distract Yourself**: To divert your attention from food cravings, engage in pleasurable activities or tasks. Play an instrument, read a book, solve puzzles, work on a creative project, or engage in other mind- and hand-occupying activities.

9. **Mindful Eating Practices**: If you do decide to eat because you're bored or under emotional stress, try mindful eating to become more conscious of the foods you choose to eat and how you eat. Savor

every bite of food, eat slowly, and be aware of your body's signals of hunger and fullness. Pick foods that will nourish you and meet your emotional and physical needs.

10. Seek Professional Assistance If Needed: If emotional stress- or boredom-induced cravings become a hindrance to your ability to control your eating patterns or general well-being, you may want to think about getting in touch with a licensed dietitian, therapist, or counselor. To assist you in navigating challenging emotions and creating healthier coping mechanisms, they can offer you individualized guidance, coping strategies, and support.

You can learn to control cravings brought on by boredom or emotional stress in a more positive and healthy way by putting these strategies into practice. Be patient with yourself as you experiment with new coping mechanisms and create healthier routines because change takes time and practice.

Part VII: Developing a Supportive Environment

The significance of social support in overcoming cravings.

Social support is extremely important in overcoming cravings and developing healthier eating habits. Here are a few reasons why social support is crucial in this process:

1. Accountability: Having supportive friends, family, or a support group can help you stay focused on your goals and resist cravings. Knowing that others believe in you and expect you to make healthier choices can help you stay on track.

2. Encouragement: When you're dealing with cravings or challenges, supportive people can offer encouragement and positive feedback. Their words of encouragement can boost your confidence and remind you of your own strengths and abilities to overcome challenges.

3. Sharing Strategies: Connecting with others who share similar goals can allow you to share effective craving-management strategies and tips. Hearing about other people's experiences and learning what worked for them can give you valuable insights and inspiration for your own journey.

4. Emotional Support: Coping with cravings and changing your eating habits can be emotionally difficult. A support system can provide a safe space for you to express your emotions, share your struggles, and receive empathy and understanding from others who have been in your situation.

5. Practical Assistance: Supportive individuals can provide practical assistance in a variety of ways, including meal planning and preparation, healthy recipe ideas, and joint participation in physical activities. Their willingness to assist others can make it easier to develop and maintain healthier habits.

6. Reduced Stress: Social support has been shown to lower stress levels, which can help manage cravings caused by stress or negative emotions. Simply knowing that you have people who care about you can help you feel less anxious and stressed.

7. Increased Confidence: Knowing that you have the support of others can boost your faith in your ability to overcome cravings and make healthier choices. Believing in yourself and your ability to change is critical for overcoming cravings and achieving your goals.

8. Celebrating Progress: Sharing milestones and accomplishments with supportive people can be extremely rewarding and motivating. Sharing your accomplishments with others can help reinforce positive behaviors, whether it's meeting a weight loss goal, resisting a particularly difficult craving, or consistently making healthier choices.

9. Sense of Belonging: Participating in a supportive community or network can give you a sense of belonging and connection, which is beneficial to your overall well-being. Knowing that you are not alone in your struggles and that others are dealing with similar issues can help you feel more connected and united.

10. Long-Term Maintenance: Social support is essential not only for overcoming cravings initially, but also for sustaining long-term success. A strong support system can help you maintain your healthier habits over time while navigating any obstacles or setbacks that may arise along the way.

Overall, social support is a valuable tool for overcoming cravings and developing healthier eating habits. Connecting with others who share your goals and values, whether through friends, family members, support groups, or online communities, can provide invaluable encouragement, guidance, and motivation as you strive for better health and well-being.

Strategies for communicating with family and friends about your goals.

When communicating with family and friends about your goals, especially those related to craving management or adopting healthier eating habits, it is critical to approach the conversation with empathy, clarity, and assertiveness. Here are some tips for effectively communicating with your loved ones about your goals:

1. Be Clear and Specific: Clearly articulate your goals and the reasons for them. Explain why you value managing cravings and adopting healthier eating habits, as well as how they align with your values

and priorities. Give specific examples of the changes you intend to make, as well as how your loved ones will help you achieve them.

2. Establish Boundaries: Be assertive in communicating your needs and boundaries with family and friends. Tell them what kind of assistance you require and what behaviors or comments are not helpful or supportive. For example, if certain foods or behaviors make you crave them, politely ask your loved ones to respect your boundaries by not bringing those items into the house or making comments that undermine your efforts.

3. Educate and Inform: Share information and resources with your family and friends to help them understand your goals and the strategies you're using to get there. Provide accurate information about the benefits of managing cravings or adopting healthier eating habits, as well as dispelling common food and nutrition myths.

4. Set a good example for your loved ones by exhibiting healthy behaviors and making wise decisions in your own life. Demonstrate to them that managing cravings and developing healthier eating habits is not only possible, but also enjoyable and rewarding. Invite them to join you in trying new recipes, preparing

healthy meals together, or engaging in physical activities that you enjoy.

5. Express Gratitude: Acknowledge and thank your family and friends for their support and encouragement. Let them know how much their encouragement means to you and how it helps you stay motivated and committed to your objectives. Positive reinforcement can strengthen your bond and encourage ongoing support.

6. Be Open to Feedback: Keep an open mind and be receptive to feedback from your loved ones, even if it's not always what you want to hear. Consider their perspectives and insights with an open

heart and mind, and be prepared to change your strategy if necessary. Remember that communication is two-way, and constructive feedback can help you grow and improve.

7. Seek Compromise: Find ways to accommodate your family and friends' needs and preferences while remaining true to your goals. Look for innovative solutions that make everyone feel heard and valued, such as finding healthier alternatives to favorite family recipes or organizing activities that help you achieve your goals while also being enjoyable for everyone.

8. Be Patient and Persistent: Changing habits and behaviors takes time, so be patient with yourself and your loved ones as you work toward your shared goals. Stay focused on your objectives and don't be discouraged by setbacks or challenges along the way. Maintain open lines of communication while advocating for your needs and priorities with kindness and persistence.

Using these strategies, you can effectively communicate your goals to your family and friends, gain their support, and create a supportive environment that promotes your success in managing cravings and adopting healthier eating habits. Remember that developing healthy habits

is a process, and having the support of
your loved ones can make all the
difference in reaching your goals.

Creating a community of accountability partners and support groups

Building a network of accountability partners and support groups can help you stay motivated, accountable, and supported as you work to manage cravings and adopt healthier eating habits. Here's how you can create such a network.

1. Find Potential Partners: Begin by identifying people in your life who have similar goals or interests in managing cravings and improving their eating habits. These could be friends, family members, coworkers, neighbors, or acquaintances who want to improve their own health and well-being.

2. Reach out: Once you've identified potential accountability partners, contact them and express your desire to form a support network. Be open and honest about your goals, challenges, and the type of assistance you're seeking. Invite them to join you on your journey, and offer to help them in return.

3. Schedule regular check-in meetings or calls with your accountability partners to share updates, discuss challenges, celebrate successes, and offer each other encouragement and support. These check-ins can help you stay on track with your goals while also providing a sense of community and support.

4. Establish Clear Goals: Clearly define and share your goals and objectives for controlling cravings and improving your eating habits with your accountability partners. Make your goals specific, measurable, achievable, relevant, and time-bound (SMART), and keep your partners up to date on your progress.

5. Foster a Supportive Environment: Within your accountability group, create a supportive and nonjudgmental environment in which members feel comfortable sharing their struggles, seeking advice, and encouraging one another. Encourage members of the group

to communicate openly, listen actively, and show empathy.

6. Share Resources and Strategies: With your accountability partners, share resources, tips, and strategies for overcoming cravings and eating healthier. This could include sharing healthy recipes, meal planning tips, mindfulness techniques, exercise routines, and other useful resources.

7. Celebrate Successes Together: Recognize each other's accomplishments, no matter how small, and the progress you've made toward your objectives. Whether you're reaching a milestone, resisting a tempting craving, or trying a

new healthy recipe, take the time to acknowledge and celebrate your accomplishments together.

8. Join Support Groups or Online Communities: In addition to creating your own accountability network, think about joining support groups or online communities that focus on craving management, healthy eating, or overall health. These groups can offer additional encouragement, support, and resources from people who have similar goals and experiences.

9. Be Flexible and Adaptive: Be adaptable in your approach to accountability partnerships and support groups.

Recognize that different people's needs, preferences, and schedules may vary, and be willing to adapt your approach to accommodate these differences.

10. Be a Supportive Partner: Finally, remember to encourage and support your accountability group members. Encourage them, recognize their efforts, and offer help and advice as needed. Supporting others on their journey will strengthen your own commitment to your own goals.

Creating a network of accountability partners and support groups can help you stay motivated, accountable, and successful in managing cravings and adopting healthier eating habits. You can celebrate your accomplishments, overcome obstacles, and strive for a healthier and happier lifestyle together.

Creating an environment that promotes healthy habits and reduces temptation.

Creating an environment that promotes healthy habits and discourages temptation is critical to your efforts to manage cravings and adopt healthier eating habits. Here are some strategies to assist you in creating such an environment.

1. Keep a variety of nutritious foods in your kitchen, such as fruits and vegetables, whole grains, lean proteins, and healthy fats. Having healthy options on hand makes it easier to make nutritious choices when cravings arise.

2. Prepare Healthy Snacks in Advance: Prepare healthy snacks ahead of time and portion them into convenient containers or

bags. Having pre-portioned snacks on hand can help you resist the urge to reach for less nutritious options when hunger strikes.

3. Limit Junk Food Purchases: To reduce the presence of junk food and highly processed snacks in your home, limit your purchases. Instead, choose whole, minimally processed foods that promote your health and well-being.

4. Keep Tempting Foods Out of Sight: Keep less healthy foods like sweets, chips, and other high-calorie snacks out of sight and reach. To reduce their visibility and accessibility, store them in less accessible locations or opaque containers.

5. Organize Your Pantry and Fridge: Keeping your pantry and fridge organized will make healthier options more visible and accessible. Arrange nutritious foods at eye level and less healthy options in less visible locations.

6. Use Smaller Plates and Bowls: To keep portion sizes under control and prevent overeating, serve meals and snacks on smaller plates and bowls. According to research, using smaller dishes can help reduce calorie intake without leaving you feeling deprived.

7. Make a Meal Plan: Plan your meals and snacks for the week ahead of time to

ensure you have nutritious options on hand. Make a grocery list based on your meal plan and purchase the ingredients you'll need to prepare healthy meals and snacks.

8. Cook at Home More Frequently: Cooking meals at home allows you to have more control over the ingredients and cooking methods used. Homemade meals are usually lower in calories, sodium, and unhealthy fats than restaurant or takeaway options.

9. Practice Mindful Eating: When eating, pay attention to your hunger and fullness cues, as well as the taste, texture, and aroma of your food. Avoid eating in front

of a television or computer because it can lead to mindless overeating.

10. Foster a Supportive Social Environment: Surround yourself with friends, family members, and coworkers who will encourage and support your efforts to adopt healthier habits. Share your goals with them and ask for their help in making positive changes.

11. Establish Healthy Routines: Develop healthy routines and habits that promote your health, such as regular exercise, adequate sleep, stress management techniques, and self-care practices. These habits can help reduce cravings while also improving overall health and well-being.

12. Practice Self-Compassion: Be kind to yourself and accept that it's okay to indulge in treats on occasion. Avoid strict rules or rigid diets, which can cause feelings of deprivation and binge eating. Rather, strive for moderation and equilibrium in your dietary practices.

By implementing these strategies, you can create an environment that encourages you to control your cravings and adopt healthier eating habits. Remember that developing healthy habits takes time and consistency, so be patient with yourself as you change your lifestyle.

Part VIII: Upkeep and Extended Prosperity

Sustaining a healthy lifestyle: the journey beyond weight loss

Maintaining a healthy lifestyle that takes mental, emotional, and physical well-being into account is the journey beyond weight loss. Beyond losing weight, follow these tips to keep up a healthy lifestyle:

1. Accept Sustainable Habits: Give special attention to forming long-term healthy and happy habits. This entails self-care routines, stress management, a healthy diet, enough sleep, and frequent physical activity.

2. Prioritize Nutrition: Keep including nutrient-dense, whole foods in your diet as a top priority. For the purpose of providing your body with necessary nutrients, try to

eat a range of fruits, vegetables, whole grains, lean proteins, and healthy fats.

3. Stay Active: Make time for regular exercise in your everyday schedule. Include enjoyable activities on a regular basis in your schedule. Walking, running, cycling, swimming, and taking part in group exercise classes are a few examples of this.

4. Listen to Your Body: Be aware of the signals your body sends about hunger and fullness as well as the feelings that particular foods elicit. You can have a healthy relationship with food if you eat mindfully and pay attention to your body's signals.

5. Manage Stress: To lessen the negative effects of stress on your general wellbeing, learn stress management strategies. This could involve practicing yoga, deep breathing techniques, mindfulness meditation, or spending time in nature.

6. Make Sleep a Priority: To maintain both physical and mental health, make sleep a priority every night. For the purpose of encouraging restful sleep, set up a regular sleep schedule, a calming bedtime ritual, and a sleep-friendly environment.

7. Foster Good Relationships: Be in the company of encouraging and motivating friends and family members. Make time

for the important relationships that give you a sense of purpose and emotional stability.

8. Exercise Self-Care: Give yourself the attention you deserve by doing things that feed your body, mind, and spirit. This could be engaging in leisure activities, learning new skills, hanging out with loved ones, or pursuing interests outside of work.

9. Create Achievable and Realistic Goals: Create attainable goals that are consistent with your priorities and values. Instead of aiming for perfection, concentrate on making small steps forward.

10. Maintain Flexibility: When it comes to leading a healthy lifestyle, be adaptable and flexible. You should be ready to modify your routines and habits when necessary because life will undoubtedly have its ups and downs.

11. Celebrate Progress: Honor your accomplishments and significant anniversaries along the road. Celebrate your efforts to keep up a healthy lifestyle and acknowledge the progress you've made.

12. Seek Assistance: Never hesitate to ask for help when you need it. Establishing a support network, comprising friends, family, and medical experts, can

significantly impact the upkeep of a healthy way of life.

You can maintain a healthy lifestyle beyond weight loss and experience long-lasting health and well-being by adopting these principles into your daily routine. Keep in mind that improving your health is a journey, and every victory is something to be proud of.

How to handle setbacks and avoid relapsing

Beyond weight loss, sustaining a healthy lifestyle also involves preventing relapse and handling setbacks. To help you stay on course and overcome setbacks, consider the following strategies:

1. Examine Patterns and Triggers: Give yourself some time to consider the things that might have led to the relapse or setback. Determine which environmental cues, social situations, stress, emotional eating, or other triggers may have affected your behavior. Your ability to identify patterns will aid in the creation of future-focused strategies.

2. Engage in Self-Compassion Practice: Show yourself kindness and compassion

when you experience failure. Recognize that obstacles to achieving improved health and wellbeing are common. Choose to be kind and understanding to yourself instead of critical or judgmental of yourself.

3. Reexamine Your Objectives: Go back to your objectives and reasons for preserving a healthy way of life. Remember the initial reasons you set out on this journey and the benefits you have gained from it. To inspire and motivate yourself to get back on track, refer to your goals.

4. Pay Attention to Progress Rather than Perfection: Reorient your attention from

perfection to forward motion. Commend yourself for your accomplishments and the constructive steps you've taken toward your goals rather than focusing on your mistakes or perceived shortcomings. Honor your accomplishments; every little step forward counts.

5. Formulate an Action Plan: To assist you in overcoming obstacles and averting relapses in the future, formulate a program of action. When faced with obstacles or triggers, know which specific coping mechanisms and strategies to employ. You can feel more in control and capable of moving forward when you have a plan in place.

Seek Assistance: During trying times, ask your network of supporters for motivation, direction, and responsibility. With family, close friends, or support groups that can provide understanding, counsel, and encouragement, discuss your problems and obstacles. In times of need, don't be embarrassed to ask for assistance.

7. Manage Stress: To properly handle stress, cultivate constructive coping strategies. This can be practicing yoga, meditation, deep breathing, or other relaxation techniques, or it could be doing relaxing and joyful activities. Emotional eating can be avoided and the chance of relapse decreased by managing stress.

8. Take Lessons from Failures: Rather than seeing setbacks as failures, see them as opportunities to learn. Give the experience some thought, and consider how you can use it to help you develop and get better. Take the opportunity presented by setbacks to reevaluate your objectives, improve your tactics, and fortify your resolve.

9. Remain Adaptive and Flexible: When it comes to upholding a healthy lifestyle, be reasonably flexible and adaptable. Being flexible with routines and strategies is important because life is full of unforeseen obstacles and changes. Try new things and be open-minded; you never know what might work better for you.

10. Appreciate Achievements: No matter how tiny, recognize and celebrate your accomplishments. It can increase your self-esteem, drive, and sense of accomplishment to recognize and celebrate small victories along the way. Admire your accomplishments and make use of them as motivation to keep going.

You can stay committed to maintaining a healthy lifestyle beyond weight loss by putting these strategies into practice, which can help you avoid relapsing and effectively manage setbacks. Remind yourself that obstacles are transitory and that you can overcome them and move closer to your objectives with perseverance, fortitude, and support.

Honoring accomplishments and establishing new objectives

In order to keep up your motivation and momentum on your journey toward a healthy lifestyle that goes beyond weight loss, it's critical to celebrate your accomplishments and set new objectives. Here's how to successfully set new goals and recognize your accomplishments:

1. Celebrate Your Success: No matter how small, take the time to celebrate and acknowledge your accomplishments. Think back on your accomplishments, the challenges you've faced, and the improvements you've witnessed. Honor your successes as a reflection of your diligence and hard work.

2. Reward Yourself: Celebrate your accomplishments by giving yourself a treat. This could be as easy as enjoying a favorite nutritious meal or engaging in a soothing self-care ritual. Select a prize that speaks to your values and demonstrates your dedication to achieving your objectives.

3. Share Your Successes: Let people who have helped you along the way know about your accomplishments. Sharing your achievements with others, whether they be friends, family, or coworkers in a support group, can uplift and encourage them and deepen your feeling of community and connection.

4. Consider Your Learnings: Give careful thought to the lessons you've drawn from your experiences and accomplishments. Think about the tactics you've found effective as well as any difficulties you've run into. Utilize these realizations to guide your future objectives and decisions.

5. Set New Objectives: To keep moving in the direction of a healthy lifestyle, after you've celebrated your successes, set new objectives. These objectives may pertain to any area of your well-being that is significant to you, such as exercise, diet, stress reduction, or sleep. Ensure that your objectives are SMART—specific, measurable, realistic, relevant, and time-bound.

6. Divide Goals into Smaller, Manageable Steps: Divide your new objectives into smaller, more doable tasks that you can accomplish gradually. You can accomplish your bigger goals by doing this, which will keep you motivated, focused, and on course. Revel in each

small victory along the road to maintain your momentum.

Remain Adaptable and Flexible: Allow yourself to modify your plans and objectives in response to new information and evolving conditions. Continue to be adaptive and flexible in your approach, and be prepared to make adjustments as you develop and learn.

8. Make a Plan of Action: To achieve your new objectives, draft a concise plan of action. Decide what specific steps you need to take, what resources you might need, and any potential roadblocks you might run into. Making a plan will assist

you in remaining focused and organized toward your goals.

9. Monitor Your Progress: To keep yourself accountable and inspired, monitor your advancement toward your new objectives. This could be using a tracking app, keeping a journal, or using a visual aid like a vision board or progress chart. To stay inspired and motivated, acknowledge and celebrate your accomplishments along the way.

10. Stay Motivated: To help you stay focused on your objectives, surround yourself with sources of inspiration and encouragement. This could involve engaging with communities that align with

your interests and aspirations, reading motivational books or articles, listening to motivational podcasts, and following positive role models on social media.

You can sustain success and fulfillment in your pursuit of a healthy lifestyle by acknowledging your accomplishments, making fresh resolutions, and remaining dedicated to your path. Recall to enjoy the process of traveling as well as the person you are evolving into.
I'll

Part IX. Conclusion.

Recap of key concepts and strategies for overcoming cravings

1. Increase mindfulness and awareness of cravings and their triggers by practicing techniques such as meditation and journaling.

2. Identification: Determine the underlying causes of cravings, which may be emotions, stress, or environmental cues.

3. Substitution: To satisfy a craving for certain foods, substitute healthier alternatives.

4. Nutritious Options: To satisfy cravings, focus on whole foods and balanced meals.

5. Variety and Creativity: Make meals and snacks more interesting and satisfying by incorporating variety and creativity.

6. Moderation: Practice moderation and balance in your eating habits, allowing yourself to indulge without guilt on occasion.

7. Social Support: Seek help from friends, family, or support groups to stay accountable and motivated.

8. Healthy Environment: Stocking up on nutritious foods can help to foster healthy habits and reduce temptation.

9.Self-Compassion: Show kindness and compassion to yourself when you experience setbacks or difficulties with craving management.

By consistently employing these strategies, you can effectively overcome cravings and maintain a healthy lifestyle.

A day's meal plan and recipe sample to aid in your travels

Breakfast: Parfait with Greek Yogurt

Ingredients: - Half a cup of plain or flavored Greek yogurt
- 1/4 cup granola, preferably low-sugar
Half a cup of mixed berries, comprising of raspberries, blueberries, and strawberries

guidelines:
1. Arrange mixed berries, granola, and Greek yogurt in a bowl or glass.
2. Continue layering until you've used every ingredient.
3. Savor this tasty and wholesome parfait as a filling option for breakfast.

Lunch is a salad made of Quinoa, chickpeas, and vegetables.

Ingredients include: - 1 cup cooked quinoa; - 1/2 cup rinsed and drained canned chickpeas; - 1 cup mixed vegetables (cherry tomatoes, bell peppers, and cucumbers).
- Two tablespoons of freshly chopped parsley, cilantro, and mint
- One tablespoon lemon juice - One tablespoon olive oil
- Season with salt and pepper.

guidelines:

1. Combine cooked quinoa, mixed vegetables, chickpeas, and finely chopped fresh herbs in a big bowl.
2. Pour the salad with lemon juice and olive oil, then toss to mix.
3. Add pepper and salt according to taste.
4. For a filling and healthy lunch option, serve cold or room temperature.

Snack: Almond butter on sliced apples

Ingredients list:
One medium apple cut into slices
– Two tsp of almond butter

1. Apply almond butter to the apple slices as directed.

2. Savor this easy and tasty snack that will keep you full in between meals with a blend of fiber, protein, and healthy fats.

Eat dinner:
Roasted Vegetables and Grilled Salmon

Four ounces of salmon filet; one cup of mixed vegetables (onions, bell peppers, zucchini, and cherry tomatoes); one tablespoon olive oil; one teaspoon lemon zest; and salt and pepper to taste

guidelines:
1. Set the grill's temperature to medium-high.
2. Add salt, pepper, and lemon zest to the salmon filet after brushing it with olive oil.

3. Put the salmon on the grill and cook it for four to five minutes on each side, or until it is well done.

4. In the meantime, combine salt, pepper, and olive oil with mixed vegetables.

5. After spreading out the vegetables on a baking sheet, roast them for 15 to 20 minutes at 400°F (200°C), or until they are soft.

6. For a tasty and nourishing supper option, serve grilled salmon with roasted veggies.

In addition to having an abundance of fruits and vegetables for fiber, vitamins, and minerals, these meal ideas offer a good ratio of protein, carbs, and healthy fats. Please feel free to modify the amounts and components to suit your specific dietary requirements and personal preferences. Savor every bite of your food!

Motivational advice

Trust Yourself: You possess the fortitude, resiliency, and willpower necessary to accomplish your weight reduction objectives. Have faith in your capacity to improve things and turn your life around.

2. Put an emphasis on Happiness and Health: Keep in mind that losing weight is about more than just a number on the scale; it's about feeling better physically, having more self-assurance, and being

happier all around. Remember the mental and physical advantages of leading a healthier lifestyle.

3. Acknowledge Every Victory: Acknowledge each little accomplishment along the road, such as shedding a few pounds, choosing better foods, or maintaining your workout schedule. Every accomplishment is an indication of your growth and a cause for celebration.

4. Focus on Each Day: Recall that losing weight is a journey rather than a sprint. Focus on making wise decisions every day and take things one day at a time. Every day presents a fresh opportunity to start, so don't let obstacles or setbacks deter you.

5. Discover Your Why: List the reasons you wish to shed pounds and make sure they are always at the front of your thoughts. A clear understanding of your "why" will help you stay motivated and laser-focused on your objectives, be they greater self-assurance, better health, or more energy to play with your children.

6. Establish a Support System: Encircle yourself with like-minded friends, relatives, or virtual networks that will uplift and motivate you during your expedition. When you most need it, having a support system in place can offer inspiration, motivation, and accountability.

7. Exercise Self-Compassion: Treat yourself with kindness as you go through your weight reduction process. Keep in mind that failures and difficult times are normal; what matters is how you handle them. Remember that you're doing your best, and be kind and understanding to yourself.

8. See Your Success: Set aside some time every day to see yourself reaching your objective of losing weight. Let your vision of yourself when you reach your goal weight encourage and inspire you to keep going. Imagine how you'll feel and look.

9. Remain Consistent: Maintaining consistency is essential for successful

weight loss. Even on the days when you don't feel like it, continue to follow your healthy habits. Never forget that every wise decision you make will get you closer to your objectives.

10. Acknowledge Your Progress: As you get closer to your weight loss objectives, stop and reflect on your accomplishments. Recognize and celebrate your victories along the road, whether they are gaining weight loss, changing the way your body looks, or experiencing better health.

Keep in mind that every person's journey to successful weight loss is different, and there will inevitably be ups and downs. Remain optimistic, committed, and believe in yourself; you can accomplish anything you set your mind to. You can succeed in this!

www.ingramcontent.com/pod-product-compliance
Lightning Source LLC
Chambersburg PA
CBHW070947250726
48663CB00002B/111